PASTEST POCK
MRCP

D0524975

BOOK 5

100 MCQs
ON
BASIC SCIENCE,
APPLIED SCIENCE
AND THERAPEUTICS

Donal J. O'Donoghue
Consultant Renal Physician
Director of Renal Medicine
Salford Royal Hospitals NHS Trust
University of Manchester

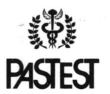

PASTEST

© 1997 PASTEST
Egerton Court, Parkgate Estate,
Knutsford, Cheshire, WA16 8DX
Telephone: 01565 755226

First edition 1997
Reprint 1998

A catalogue record for this book is available from the British Library.

ISBN: 0 906896 93 2

The information contained within this book was obtained by the author
from reliable sources. However, while every effort has been made to
ensure its accuracy, no responsibility for loss, damage or injury
occasioned to any person acting or refraining from action as a result of
information contained herein can be accepted by the publishers or
authors.

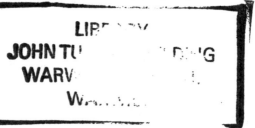
Typeset by Breeze Limited, Manchester
Printed by Bookmag, Inverness

CONTENTS

PASTEST REVISION BOOKS FOR MRCP 1

PasTest publish a wide range of revision books including:

MCQs in Basic Medical Sciences for MRCP 1
300 exam-based MCQs with answers and detailed explanatory notes

MRCP 1 Practice Exams: 2nd edition
Five complete MCQ Papers (300 MCQs) covering favourite Royal College topics

MRCP 1 MCQ Revision Book: 3rd edition
300 MCQs arranged by subject with correct answers and teaching notes, plus one complete mock exam

MRCP 1 Past Topics: A Revision Syllabus: 2nd edition
Contains authoritative lists of past topics which have occurred in the Royal College examination over the past 5 years

Explanations to the RCP Past Papers
Correct answers and teaching notes related to the Royal College Green and Blue books of actual past exam questions

MRCP Part 1 MCQs with Key Topic Summaries: 2nd edition
200 MCQs related to current examination syllabus with 200 comprehensive topic summaries

Membership at your Fingertips: MCQs on Disk
The disk contains 650 MCQs. Clear and concise teaching notes with every question

Oxford Textbook of Medicine MCQs: 3rd edition
375 new MCQs related to the 1995 Oxford Textbook of Medicine and ideal for subject based revision

For full details of all our revision books contact PasTest today on **01565 755226** for a free copy of our current book catalogue and price list. Books sent by return of post worldwide.

For full details contact:
**PasTest, Egerton Court, Parkgate Estate,
Knutsford, Cheshire WA16 8DX
Telephone 01565 755226 Fax 01565 650264**

INTRODUCTION

PasTest's MRCP Part 1 Pocket Books are designed to help the busy examination candidate to make the most of every opportunity to revise. With this little book in your pocket, it is the work of a moment to open it, choose a question, decide upon your answers and then check the answer on the back of the page. Revising 'on the run' in this manner is both reassuring (if your answer is correct) and stimulating (if you find any gaps in your knowledge).

Each book contains 100 exam-based MCQs arranged by subject. Each author is a subject specialist who has based his selection of questions on past Royal College papers, and questions have also been designed specifically to address the basic science topics that have increasing prominence in the examination.

Each question consists of an initial statement followed by five possible completions, ABCDE. There is no restriction on the number of true or false items in a question. It is possible for all items in a question to be true or for all to be false. The four most important points of technique are:

1. Read the question carefully and be sure you understand it.
2. Mark your response clearly, correctly and accurately.
3. Use reasoning to work out your answer, but if you do not know the answer and cannot work it out, indicate 'don't know'.
4. The best possible way to obtain a good mark is to have as wide a knowledge as possible of the topics being tested in the examination.

It is possible to improve your mark by educated guessing, but this must be done with great care as incorrect answers are given a mark of –1 in the exam. You can use the books in this series to work out whether or not you are a good guesser by making a special mark against the responses that you have guessed before you check whether your responses are correct.

To get the best value from this book you should commit yourself to an answer for each item before you check the correct answer. With the answers on the back of each page, it can be tempting to find out which answers are correct before you have really decided on your own answer. But it is only by being sure of your own responses that you can ascertain which questions you would find difficult in the examination. Use the check boxes to mark your answers, or mark the parts of a question that you found difficult so that next time you look at the question you will be able to home in on your own personal areas of difficulty.

Books like the ones in this series, which consist of MCQs in subject categories, can help you to home in on specific topics and to isolate your weaknesses. You should plan a revision timetable to help you spread your time fairly over the range of subjects likely to appear in the examination. PasTest's *MRCP Part 1 Past Topics: A Revision Syllabus* will help you to work out which subjects deserve most of your revision time.

An effective revision plan should also include opportunities to practise your exam technique. Books of MCQ Practice Exams are indispensable and you should make time to sit at least two or three complete practice papers under timed conditions before the day of the actual examination arrives.

PasTest Revision Courses for MRCP 1
For 25 years PasTest, the leading independent specialists in post-graduate medical education, have been delivering top quality courses that have helped many thousands of doctors to pass the demanding MRCP Part 1 examination.

Our six-day MRCP Part 1 revision courses run three times each year at a convenient central London venue. Each delegate receives detailed course notes consisting of approximately 250 pages of exam-based MCQs with answers and comprehensive notes, plus many explanatory handouts.

>   ✓ Learn from experienced and talented tutors with up-to-date knowledge of the requirements of the exam

>   ✓ Teaching sessions focus on 'favourite' exam topics and highlight possible areas of difficulty

>   ✓ Four full practice exams enable you to monitor your performance constantly as the course progresses

For full details of the range of PasTest books and courses available for MRCP Part 1 candidates, contact PasTest today:

**PasTest, Egerton Court, Parkgate Estate,
Knutsford, Cheshire WA16 8DX
Telephone: 01565 755226 Fax: 01565 650264**

CARDIOVASCULAR MEDICINE

Mark your answers with a tick (True) or a cross (False) in the box provided. Leave the box blank for 'Don't know'.

1. In the cardiac cycle

☐ A isovolumetric contraction occurs after the 2nd heart sound

☐ B the venous C wave occurs during ventricular contraction

☐ C the rate of ventricular filling increases throughout diastole

☐ D mean left ventricular pressure equals mean aortic pressure

☐ E during inspiration ventricular ejection is prolonged

2. 3–hydroxy–3–methyl glutaryl–CoA (HMGCoA) reductase inhibitors

☐ A can cause gout

☐ B increase HDL cholesterol

☐ C preferentially reduce triglycerides

☐ D can cause myositis

☐ E increase insulin sensitivity

3. Losartan

☐ A is a specific renal angiotensin converting enzyme inhibitor

☐ B induces cough in only approximately 5% of patients

☐ C can be used safely in renal artery stenosis

☐ D may exacerbate hyperkalaemia

☐ E reduces angiotensin II levels in the efferent renal arteriole

4. In pregnancy, cardiovascular changes include

☐ A an increase in pulmonary vascular resistance

☐ B an increase in blood volume of about 40%

☐ C tachycardia

☐ D an increase in cardiac output by about 45%

☐ E no change in stroke volume

Answers overleaf

1. B E

Isovolumetric contraction occurs after mitral valve closure (1st heart sound) and before aortic valve opening. Left ventricular pressure increases from 8 mmHg to 130 mmHg but in the aorta elastic recoil maintains pressure during diastole so that aortic pressure is approximately 130/75 (mean 100 mmHg). The venous C wave is due to bulging of the tricuspid valve during ventricular contraction. Ventricular filling is most rapid immediately after the A-V valves open but is augmented by atrial systole. During inspiration the ventricular ejection period is prolonged due to increased stroke volume secondary to increased venous return.

2. B D

3-hydroxy-3-methyl glutaryl-CoA (HMGCoA) reductase inhibitors inhibit cholesterol biosynthesis and can decrease serum LDL by 30–40%. Serum triglycerides are also reduced but to a much lesser extent and HDL is increased. Myositis can occur in up to 0.5% of patients. Fibric acid derivatives, but not statins, tend to produce improvement in glucose tolerance (especially bezafibrate) and fenofibrate reduces urate levels by a direct renal uricosuric action.

3. D

Losartan is an angiotensin II receptor blocker. It leads to an increase in angiotensin II. It specifically blocks the renin–angiotensin system and unlike ACE inhibitors does not increase bradykinin which has been implicated in both ACE I induced cough and angioneurotic oedema. It does however share with ACE I the side effects related to renin–angiotensin system blockade including risk of acute renal failure in renal artery stenosis and hyperkalaemia.

4. B C D

In pregnancy, peripheral and pulmonary vascular resistance fall and blood volume increases by about 40% at 30 weeks. There is an increase in the volume of plasma and in the number of red cells but the disproportionate increase in plasma leads to haemodilution. Cardiac output increases to about 45% above normal levels at 20 weeks. The increase in cardiac output is due to an increased heart rate and to larger stroke volume.

5. **Hypertrophic cardiomyopathy**
   - ☐ A is an autosomal recessive disease
   - ☐ B penetrance is uniform within defined pedigrees
   - ☐ C can result from beta myosin heavy chain gene mutations
   - ☐ D is associated with sudden death in young adults
   - ☐ E can result from several different mutations

6. **Endothelin–I**
   - ☐ A acts as a local paracrine factor
   - ☐ B vasodilates the pulmonary vasculature
   - ☐ C is elevated in heart failure
   - ☐ D is generated by a converting enzyme
   - ☐ E acts on endothelial type B receptors to promote nitric oxide production

7. **Constitutive nitric oxide synthase**
   - ☐ A is present in endothelial cells
   - ☐ B is calcium independent
   - ☐ C produces higher concentrations of nitric oxide than inducible nitric oxide synthase
   - ☐ D is not active under normal physiological conditions
   - ☐ E acts on citrulline to produce nitric oxide

Answers overleaf

5. C D

Familial hypertrophic cardiomyopathy is an autosomal dominant disease resulting in increased left ventricular mass. Its penetrance is highly variable, even within a single pedigree. The disease was first linked to a mis-sense mutation in a gene encoding a major sarcomeric protein, the beta myosin heavy chain. Subsequently mutations in different genes encoding other sarcomeric proteins have been identified that can cause the hypertrophic cardiomyopathy phenotype. The clinical course of hypertrophic cardiomyopathy is highly variable – features can include arrhythmias, mural thrombi and embolic events, infective endocarditis, cardiac failure and syncope or sudden death in previously asymptomatic children and young adults.

6. A C D E

Endothelin–I is an endothelium-derived vasoconstrictor and pressor peptide with mitogenic properties that is generated from a precursor, 'big' endothelin–I, through the action of endothelin converting enzyme (that is distinct from angiotensin converting enzyme). Endothelin–I is present in plasma but it is mainly released towards smooth muscle and acts in a paracrine fashion. It is elevated in heart failure, vasospasm and acute renal failure. Endothelin–I acts on type A receptors in smooth muscle to cause vasoconstriction. Type B receptors are on endothelial cells and modulate vasoconstriction by generation of the vasodilators, nitric oxide and prostacyclin.

7. A

Constitutive nitric oxide synthase is present in endothelial cells and requires a rise in cytosolic free calcium for activation. Stimulation of the constitutive nitric oxide synthase generates nitric oxide of picomolar concentrations, while the amount of nitric oxide produced by the inducible enzyme, after exposure to endotoxin and cytokines is much greater. The inducible nitric oxide synthase is calcium independent. Inhibition of constitutive nitric oxide synthase causes a rise in blood pressure demonstrating that basal nitric oxide production by endothelial cells is physiologically important in blood flow regulation. Nitric oxide is produced from arginine not citrulline.

8. Homocystinuria

- ☐ A is associated with aortic dilation
- ☐ B pyridoxine does not reduce homocystine levels but does improve symptoms
- ☐ C is an X–linked disorder
- ☐ D can be treated with penicillamine
- ☐ E causes renal stones

9. Sotalol

- ☐ A has intrinsic sympathomimetic activity
- ☐ B is a selective beta-adrenoreceptor antagonist
- ☐ C prolongs the QT interval
- ☐ D is metabolised by the liver
- ☐ E should be avoided in paroxysmal atrial fibrillation

10. Concerning cardiac sarcomere

- ☐ A contraction is calcium dependent
- ☐ B tropomyosin is a component of the thick filaments
- ☐ C relaxation is ATP dependent
- ☐ D troponin I inhibits the interaction between actin and myosin
- ☐ E the thin filament is made of actin

Answers overleaf

8. None correct

Homocystinuria is an autosomal recessive disorder due to deficiency of beta-cystathione synthetase. It shares many phenotypic features with Marfan's syndrome but patients do not develop aortic root dilation. There is an increased arterial thrombotic risk. In approximately 50% of patients homocystine levels (and thrombotic risk) fall with pyridoxine therapy. It does not cause renal stones. Urinary cystine stones can be treated by penicillamine which increases the solubility of cystine in urine (but does not alter urinary cystine concentration).

9. C

Sotalol is a competitive, non-selective beta-adrenoreceptor antagonist which is devoid of intrinsic sympathomimetic activity. It has class III antiarrythmic properties, prolonging both atrial and ventricular action potential duration and refractory periods. It is useful in terminating, and for prophylaxis of, atrial flutter, atrial fibrillation and ventricular ectopics/tachycardia. It does prolong the QT interval and increases the risk of torsade de pointes – post myocardial infarction it has been associated with increased mortality. It is not metabolised by the liver but is excreted unchanged by the kidneys and accumulates in renal failure.

10. A C D E

The sarcomere is made of two interdigitating filaments, thick filaments of myosin and thin filaments of actin. The actin filaments have a complex structure associated with tropomyosin which maintains the structure of the actin chain and troponin complex. Contraction in the cardiac sarcomere is initiated by the binding of calcium to troponin C which then no longer causes troponin I to inhibit the interaction between actin and myosin. The myosin head contains an ATPase which breaks down ATP to provide energy for contraction but ATP is also necessary for relaxation.

Mark your answers with a tick (True) or a cross (False) in the box provided. Leave the box blank for 'Don't know'.

11. Cystic fibrosis

☐ A phenotype correlates with cystic fibrosis transmembrane regulator function

☐ B is associated with obstructive azoospermia

☐ C results from a single mutation to the cystic fibrosis transmembrane conductance regulator gene

☐ D is inherited in an autosomal dominant fashion

☐ E can be excluded if genotyping is normal

12. Physiological factors that increase the P50 of haemoglobin – O_2 include

☐ A increase in hydrogen ion concentration

☐ B reduction in pCO_2

☐ C increase in temperature

☐ D increase in 2,3 diphosphoglycerate (2,3 DPG)

☐ E reduced chloride ion concentration

13. Allergic bronchopulmonary aspergillosis

☐ A is associated with eosinophilia

☐ B usually occurs in patients with chronic asthma

☐ C antibodies to *Aspergillus* can be detected in serum

☐ D *Aspergillus* antigen skin testing is rarely positive

☐ E is a form of extrinsic allergic alveolitis

Answers overleaf

11. A B

Cystic fibrosis is an autosomal recessive disease caused by mutations to the cystic fibrosis transmembrane conductance regulator (CFTR) genes on chromosome 7. Both genes must be affected for cystic fibrosis to develop. Over 500 CFTR mutations associated with cystic fibrosis are known. Genotyping can therefore be difficult to interpret — failure to find two abnormal genes does not rule out the disease. In about 1% of those with the disease no abnormal gene can be found and in about 18% more only one abnormal gene will be identified. Even if both genes are abnormal, the individual may not have the disease because some mutations ameliorate or neutralise the primary mutation. There is a close correlation between phenotype (clinical manifestations) and the percentage of normal CFTR function: <1% severe disease and pancreatic failure; <5% pulmonary disease; <10% congenital absence of the vas deferens; >10% no abnormality.

12. A C D

The P50 of haemoglobin is the partial pressure of oxygen at which half the haemoglobin is oxygenated. Factors that increase the P50 will shift the haemoglobin–oxygen curve to the right releasing more O_2 to the tissues, i.e. an increased P50 reflects reduced oxygen affinity. The effect of acidosis on the oxygen affinity of haemoglobin is known as the Bohr effect. Temperature and 2,3 DPG also directly increase P50. Carbon dioxide has a minor effect on oxygen affinity — also shifting the curve to the right. Chloride ions do not have a direct effect on oxygen affinity but do increase in acidosis (the chloride shift) because of the free diffusion of HCO_3 ions out of erythrocytes.

13. A B C

Allergic bronchopulmonary aspergillosis typically occurs in chronic asthmatics. Inhaled *Aspergillus fumigatus* spores germinate and grow in bronchi triggering antibody production and eosinophilia. Identification of fungal hyphae in casts is diagnostic, but skin tests are also positive in 90% of cases. Bronchopulmonary aspergillosis is not a form of extrinsic allergic alveolitis, although *Aspergillus clavatus* can cause allergic alveolitis in malt workers.

14. In non small cell lung cancer

- ☐ A over expression of the ras oncogene is associated with poor progress
- ☐ B proliferating cell nuclear antigen expression is inversely correlated with survival
- ☐ C outcome is independent of the Karnowsky Scale
- ☐ D adjuvant chemotherapy is superior if histology is non-squamous
- ☐ E the relative risks of combined exposure to asbestos and cigarette smoking are not additive

15. In sarcoidosis

- ☐ A T cells accumulate in active lesions
- ☐ B granulomas caseate
- ☐ C CD4 +ve helper T cells are increased in peripheral blood
- ☐ D there is B cell overactivity
- ☐ E activated pulmonary macrophages produce calcitriol

16. Alpha-1-antitrypsin deficiency

- ☐ A is associated with systemic vasculitis
- ☐ B does not cause emphysema in non-smokers
- ☐ C heterozygotes are unaffected
- ☐ D is associated with neonatal hepatitis in only 10% of individuals
- ☐ E affects 1% of the UK population

Answers overleaf

14. A B

Molecular genetic markers of prognosis in non small cell lung cancer include the ras oncogene and p21 expression. The ras oncogenes modulate cell growth via regulation of the signal transduction pathway. Ras genes are expressed in virtually all cells, but mutations can lead to over expression and increased production of P21, the protein product of Ras – this is associated with poor outcome. Proliferating cell nuclear antigen, a nuclear protein that binds to DNA polymerase and can be used as a marker of cell proliferation, is also associated with poor outcome. Karnowsky performance status, extent of disease and weight loss are the most powerful determinants of survival. Histological type does not affect response to adjuvant chemotherapy. The risks of smoking (relative risk increased by 11) and asbestos (relative risk increased by 6) exposure are multiplicative (relative risk increased by 59).

15. A D E

Sarcoidosis is a multisystem disorder of unknown aetiology characterised by accumulation of T cells, monocytes and non-caseating granulomas in involved tissues. Bronchopulmonary lavage usually reveals lymphocytic pleocytosis with a predominance of CD4 +ve T cells. In comparison to the BAL findings, the peripheral blood of patients with pulmonary sarcoidosis shows a T cell lymphopenia due to reduced CD4 +ve T cells. There is also generalised B cell hyperactivity with hypergammaglobulinaemia. The hypercalcaemia of sarcoidosis is secondary to elevated calcitriol secreted by activated pulmonary macrophages.

16. A C D

Alpha-1-antitrypsin is a serum protease inhibitor and levels are controlled by a polymorphic system with multiple alleles. The homozygous ZZ genotype is associated with emphysema, neonatal and adult hepatitis/cirrhosis and systemic vasculitis. In smokers symptoms of emphysema are present earlier and are more severe. Heterozygotes of the MZ and MS genotypes have normal or only marginally reduced alpha-1-antitrypsin levels and are not predisposed to emphysema. Neonatal hepatitis affects about 10% of ZZ homozygotes – it is assumed that an environmental trigger in addition to the deficiency is required for this manifestation. The frequency of alpha-1-antitrypsin deficiency is about 0.05%.

17. Hyperventilation is a feature of

- ☐ A brain stem dsyfunction
- ☐ B metabolic acidosis
- ☐ C pyrexia
- ☐ D salicylate poisoning
- ☐ E hypocapnia

18. The physiological adaptations to high altitude living include

- ☐ A development of a mild systemic acidosis
- ☐ B reduced renal excretion of bicarbonate
- ☐ C reduced red cell 2,3 diphosphoglycerate (2,3 DPG)
- ☐ D no change in circulating blood volume
- ☐ E pulmonary hypertension

19. In respiratory function tests

- ☐ A residual volume is reduced in chronic bronchitis
- ☐ B total lung capacity is reduced in farmers' lung
- ☐ C arterial PO_2 is a good predictor of respiratory failure in Guillain–Barré syndrome
- ☐ D transfer factor is normal in lymphangitis carcinomatosis
- ☐ E inspiratory flow is more affected than expiratory flow if large airway obstruction is intrathoracic

Answers overleaf

17. A B C D

Hypercapnia is the strongest stimulus to breathing by the action of carbon dioxide on the central chemoreceptors. Increased hydrogen ion concentration will also activate the central chemoreceptors in metabolic acidosis resulting in Kussmaul's respiration. The hyperventilatory response to fever is probably mediated by a central effect of raised interleukins. Aspirin also directly stimulates the respiratory centres and poisoning results in a complex acid base disturbance with mixed metabolic acidosis and respiratory alkalosis. Sustained rapid and deep ventilation often occurs following brain stem tegmentum injury.

18. E

The response to chronic hypoxia (e.g. high altitude acclimatization) includes increased ventilation which reduces carbon dioxide levels and causes a mild alkalosis that is corrected by increased renal bicarbonate excretion. Red cell 2,3 DPG is increased facilitating shift of the $Hb\text{-}O_2$ dissociation curve to the right. Haemoglobin concentration and circulating blood volume increase and there is pulmonary hypertension due to pulmonary vasoconstriction caused by chronic hypoxia.

19. B

In chronic bronchitis the vital capacity and total lung capacity fall, but residual volume is increased because of chest overexpansion. In interstitial lung diseases such as cryptogenic fibrosing alveolitis, extrinsic allergic alveolitis (e.g. farmers' lung) and lymphangitis carcinomatosis the major features are significantly reduced lung volumes and impaired transfer factor. Flow volume loops can distinguish intra from extra-thoracic obstruction because large airway intrathoracic obstruction affects expiration more than inspiration. In neuromuscular disease, such as Guillain–Barré syndrome, arterial PO_2 is a poor predictor of subsequent respiratory failure – a falling PEFR is a much better predictor.

20. Concerning type I and type II pneumocytes

☐ A type I pneumocytes are more numerous than type II cells

☐ B type I pneumocytes predominantly provide the epithelial lining of the alveoli

☐ C type II pneumocytes produce surfactant

☐ D type II pneumocytes have phagocyte capacity

☐ E only type I pneumocytes are ciliated

Answers overleaf

20. B C D

Type II pneumocytes are slightly more numerous than type I cells, but cover less of the epithelial lining. The type I cells have an extremely attenuated cytoplasm and thus only provide a thin barrier to gas exchange across the alveolar membrane. They are derived from type II pneumocytes. In contrast, type II pneumocytes are more cuboidal in shape and cover a more limited surface area. The principal physiological activity of type II pneumocytes is production of surfactant but they also have limited phagocytic ability. Surfactant is an insoluble liproprotein largely consisting of dipalmitoyl lecithin which lowers the surface tension in the alveoli. Cilia only extend to the respiratory bronchiole; neither pneumocyte is ciliated.

Mark your answers with a tick (True) or a cross (False) in the box provided. Leave the box blank for 'Don't know'.

21. Factor V Leiden

□ A results in enhanced sensitivity to protein C

□ B occurs due to a premature stop codon in the gene for factor V

□ C venous thromboembolic risk is only increased in homozygotes

□ D is an acquired defect

□ E is associated with recurrent abortion

22. Vitamin B12

□ A is absorbed in the ileum

□ B requirements are increased in lead poisoning

□ C is a co-enzyme in red cell membrane synthesis

□ D is transported by intrinsic factor to the bone marrow

□ E deficiency is associated with gastric carcinoid formation

23. Glucose-6-phosphate dehydrogenase deficiency

□ A is an autosomal recessive condition

□ B provides protection against *Plasmodium falciparum*

□ C haemolysis can be precipitated by chloroquine

□ D haemoglobin electrophoresis is normal

□ E results in osmotic fragility

Answers overleaf

21. None correct

Factor V Leiden results from a single amino acid substitution at position 506 of glutamine for arginine. The resultant factor V in its activated form is resistant to cleavage by the natural anticoagulant protein C. Venous thromboembolism develops in up to 40% of heterozygotes and heterozygotes account for about 15% of all thromboembolic episodes. The condition is hereditary. Unlike the antiphospholipid antibodies syndrome it is not associated with recurrent abortion.

22. A E

Vitamin B12 in animal food binds to a glycoprotein – intrinsic factor – which is secreted by parietal cells in the stomach and is absorbed via a specific receptor on the surface of the mucosa of the ileum. Vitamin B12 enters the ileal cells and intrinsic factor remains in the lumen. Vitamin B12, like folate, is a key enzyme in the synthesis of DNA – deficiency of either reduces the availability of methylene tetrahydrofolate polyglutamate. Lead poisoning interferes with haem and globin synthesis resulting in abnormal erythrocytes with basophilic stippling. In pernicious anaemia there is atrophy of the gastric mucosa, achlorhydria and increased risk of both gastric carcinoids and gastric carcinoma.

23. B C D

Glucose-6-phosphate dehydrogenase (G6PD) is a vital enzyme in the hexose monophosphate pathway that provides glutathione in a reduced state for the red cell. Glutathione reduces oxidative stress on the red cell, maintaining membrane flexibility and avoiding oxidation of haemoglobin that would result in methaemoglobin formation. G6PD deficiency is sex linked. Deficiency of the enzyme provides protection against *Plasmodium falciparum*. Attacks of acute haemolysis are usually precipitated by drugs or infection. Haemoglobin electrophoresis is normal as is osmotic fragility.

24. Haemopoietin growth factors

- ☐ A act on colony forming units
- ☐ B include interleukin-3
- ☐ C are members of the immunoglobulin superfamily
- ☐ D are encoded for by genes on chromosome 3
- ☐ E do not affect mature cell function

25. Antiphospholipid antibodies

- ☐ A are monoclonal
- ☐ B are associated with recurrent abortion
- ☐ C cause a bleeding diathesis
- ☐ D interfere with the Wasserman reaction
- ☐ E clinical manifestations include Addison's disease

26. Sézary syndrome

- ☐ A has an excellent prognosis
- ☐ B is a B cell malignancy
- ☐ C frequently evolves into a non-Hodgkin's lymphoma
- ☐ D often presents with generalised erythroderma
- ☐ E lymphocytes have a typical hairy appearance

27. Warfarin

- ☐ A inhibits vitamin K independent coagulation factors
- ☐ B increases levels of the coagulation inhibitor protein C
- ☐ C causes microscopic haematuria
- ☐ D is teratogenic
- ☐ E metabolism is inhibited by rifampicin

Answers overleaf

24. A B

The haemopoietic growth factors are glycoprotein hormones that regulate the proliferation and differentiation of haemopoietic progenitor cells and the function of mature cells. They include erythropoietin, granulocyte macrophage colony stimulating factor (GM-CSF), granulocyte colony stimulating factor (G-CSF), macrophage colony stimulating factor (M-CSF) and interleukin-3. Each growth factor is encoded by a single gene on a number of different chromosomes. These factors are unrelated to the immunoglobulin superfamily.

25. B D E

Antiphospholipid antibodies are a heterogeneous population of immunoglobulins directed against cardiolipin and beta 2 glycoprotein I (B2-GPI). These autoantibodies interfere with the Wasserman reaction giving a so called biological false–positive serological test for syphilis. *In vitro* they also interfere with the activated partial thromboplastin time and are termed lupus anticoagulant but *in vivo*, paradoxically, lead to increased thrombotic risk including placental thrombosis resulting in recurrent abortion and adrenal gland thrombotic infarction.

26. C D

Sézary syndrome is part of a spectrum of T cell malignancies which often involve the skin in a diffuse erythrodermic reaction. The cells are large, cleaved, mononuclear cells distinct from the small spiky (or hairy) cells of hairy cell leukaemia. Immunological markers have shown these cells to be helper T cells in origin. The prognosis is poor, most patients die within a few years, often from a non-Hodgkin's lymphoma.

27. D

The anticoagulant effect of warfarin is mediated by the inhibition of the vitamin K dependent gamma-carboxylation of coagulation factors II, VII, IX and X. Warfarin also inhibits vitamin K-dependent gamma carboxylation of the coagulation inhibitors protein C and protein S. Anticoagulation does not cause haematuria unless there is an associated renal or genitourinary tract lesion. Warfarin is contra-indicated in pregnancy because it is teratogenic. Warfarin is heavily protein bound and metabolised by cytochrome P450 – it is therefore susceptible to many drug interactions including increased metabolism when administered in conjunction with the enzyme inducer rifampicin.

28. Paroxysmal nocturnal haemoglobinuria

- ☐ A is exacerbated by alkalosis
- ☐ B is due to a deficiency of red cell membrane bound decay accelerating factor
- ☐ C is an inherited haemoglobinopathy
- ☐ D can present as the Budd–Chiari syndrome
- ☐ E is associated with leukaemia

29. Plasma exchange has been shown to be beneficial in

- ☐ A Guillian–Barré syndrome
- ☐ B rheumatoid arthritis
- ☐ C membranous nephropathy
- ☐ D acute allograft rejection
- ☐ E Waldenström's macroglobulinaemia

30. Cold autoimmune haemolytic anaemia

- ☐ A has a peak incidence above 60 years
- ☐ B antibodies are typically IgG
- ☐ C causes intravascular haemolysis
- ☐ D antibodies are directed to the I-antigen
- ☐ E is secondary to cryoglobulinaemia

Answers overleaf

28. B D E

Paroxysmal nocturnal haemoglobinuria (PNH) is an acquired genetic disorder of the glycosyl-phosphatidyl-inositol anchor that binds the complement neutralising protein decay accelerating factor to the red cell membrane. The result is increased red cell sensitivity to complement lysis. This is exacerbated by acidosis – explaining the nocturnal nature of haemolysis – and is the basis for Ham's acid lysis test. PNH results in thrombotic events such as hepatic vein thrombosis and is associated with aplastic anaemia and a number of leukaemias.

29. A E

Plasma exchange involves the withdrawal of blood, removal of plasma and the return to the patient of the red cell enriched fraction plus donor plasma. Benefits may arise from removal of mediators of tissue damage, replacement of deficient factors or immunomodulating effects of human immunoglobin. Although plasma exchange has been used in many instances of presumed immune mediated disease, clear benefit is only apparent in a few. In severe Guillian–Barré syndrome, plasma exchange or immunoglobulin infusion is beneficial. Acute allograft rejection is a cell mediated phenomenon and is not responsive to plasma exchange. Plasma exchange is useful in the emergency treatment of hyperviscosity syndrome due to, for example, Waldenström's macroglobulinaemia, myeloma, cold agglutinin disease or cryoglobulinaemia.

30. A C D

Cold autoimmune haemolytic anaemia is a disorder of the elderly. Secondary cases occasionally occur in association with non-Hodgkin's lymphoma, *Mycoplasma pneumoniae* or infectious mononucleosis. The red cells become coated with IgM antibodies to the I-antigen in the patient's cold extremities. As the blood warms, complement is activated and intravascular haemolysis occurs. Cryoglobulins are immunoglobulins which form precipitates in the cold – they are distinct from cold agglutinins.

Mark your answers with a tick (True) or a cross (False) in the box provided. Leave the box blank for 'Don't know'.

31. The following cause resistance to erythropoietin treatment of renal anaemia:

- ☐ A iron deficiency
- ☐ B infection
- ☐ C antibodies to erythropoietin
- ☐ D hyperparathyroidism
- ☐ E angiotensin converting enzyme inhibitors

32. The following drugs accumulate if renal function is impaired:

- ☐ A tobramycin
- ☐ B simvastatin
- ☐ C acyclovir
- ☐ D allopurinol
- ☐ E nifedipine

33. Low dose (renal dose) dopamine

- ☐ A improves renal perfusion in healthy humans
- ☐ B results in a natriuresis
- ☐ C improves renal function in established acute renal failure
- ☐ D can be associated with bowel ischaemia
- ☐ E does not result in arrhythmias

Answers overleaf

31. A B D

Erythropoietin is used for the treatment of anaemia in renal failure after non-renal causes of anaemia (e.g. bone marrow infiltration, gastrointestinal blood loss and folate/B12 deficiency) have been excluded. Any alternative cause of anaemia such as iron deficiency can lead to resistance to erythropoietin and the need for higher doses of erythropoietin to achieve satisfactory haemoglobin responses. Acute infection and chronic infections (e.g. TB or osteomyelitis) are also associated with poor response to erythropoietin by mechanisms related to increased inflammatory cytokines. Hyperparathyroidism also impairs the bone marrow response to erythropoietin. Antibodies to erythropoietin have not been detected. ACE inhibitors do not affect the response to erythropoetin.

32. A C D

The elimination of many drugs is dependent on renal excretion. Tobramycin, acyclovir and allopurinol all accumulate to toxic levels if given at standard dose for normal renal function. Aminoglycosides result in ototoxicity and renal toxicity, acyclovir can cause a toxic encephalopathy that can lead to diagnostic confusion with herpes encephalitis and allopurinol and its metabolite oxypurinol increase the risk of a serious desquamative skin eruption in renal failure. Simvastatin and nifedipine must be used with caution in hepatic impairment.

33. A B D

Renal dose dopamine augments renal blood flow, glomerular filtration and natriuresis in healthy humans. It does not, however, improve renal function or outcome in acute renal failure and has not been demonstrated to protect high risk patients. Its use in these situations is therefore controversial. Renal dose dopamine can precipitate serious cardiovascular and metabolic complications in critically ill patients, including bowel ischaemia.

34. Autosomal dominant polycystic kidney disease

☐ A has a gene frequency of 1 in 10,000

☐ B is associated with polycythaemia

☐ C usually causes end stage renal disease by the age of 40

☐ D is due to an abnormality in polycystin

☐ E liver involvement is more frequent in females

35. Vasopressin

☐ A reduces water permeability of the collecting ducts

☐ B increases urine osmolality

☐ C is elevated in nephrotic syndrome

☐ D acts via cyclic GMP

☐ E increases aquaporin expression

36. Von Hippel–Lindau disease

☐ A is associated with multifocal renal cell cancer

☐ B is autosomal recessive

☐ C is due to the loss of a tumour suppressor gene

☐ D is associated with phaeochromocytomas

☐ E is associated with retinoblastoma

Answers overleaf

34. B D E

Autosomal dominant polycystic kidney disease is common with a gene frequency of approximately 1 in 1000. Cysts can be present from birth and enlarge over time. End stage renal disease is unusual before age 40 (< 5%). The renal cysts produce excessive amounts of erythropoietin that can result in polycythaemia. Other common features are haematuria, hypertension, mitral valve prolapse and ruptured berry aneurysms. The commonest form of APCKD – type I – which accounts for 90% of cases results from an abnormality in the gene for polycystin on chromosome 16, a protein that has a role in epithelial cell differentiation. Liver cysts are more numerous and larger in women than in men, presumably as a consequence of hormonal differences.

35. B C E

The water permeability of the collecting duct is significantly increased by vasopressin, which is attained by the insertion of aquaporin water channels in endosomes into the apical membrane of the collecting ducts. This results in an increased concentration of urine. This is a cyclic AMP mediated effect (not cyclic GMP). Vasopressin is elevated during volume depletion and when the effective circulating volume is reduced as in heart failure, nephrotic syndrome and liver failure.

36. A C D

Von Hippel–Lindau (VHL) disease is an autosomal dominant disorder characterised by CNS haemangioblastoma formation, phaeochromo-cytoma, renal tumours and pancreatic tumours and cysts. The VHL gene is on the short arm of chromosome 3 and normally functions as a tumour suppressor gene. In VHL disease the gene is mutated or deleted. Retinoblastomas are due to the loss of a different tumour suppressor gene on chromosome 13.

37. The anion gap

- ☐ A is reduced in maple syrup urine disease
- ☐ B is elevated in ureterosigmoidostomy
- ☐ C is elevated in hyponatraemia
- ☐ D is reduced in the nephrotic syndrome
- ☐ E is elevated in salicylate poisoning

38. Alport's syndrome

- ☐ A is an X-linked dominant condition
- ☐ B is due to a mutation of the type III collagen gene
- ☐ C is associated with retinitis pigmentosa
- ☐ D post transplant antiglomerular basement membrane nephritis develops in 50% of patients
- ☐ E is associated with cardiac conduction abnormalities

39. Dialysis-related amyloidosis

- ☐ A results from beta 2 microglobulin deposition
- ☐ B does not occur in patients managed by peritoneal dialysis
- ☐ C can result in renal transplant failure
- ☐ D frequently presents as carpal tunnel syndrome
- ☐ E is more frequent in patients with diabetes

Answers overleaf

37. D E

The anion gap is the sum of

$(Na^+ + K^+) - (Cl^- + HCO_3)$

It is normally between 10 and 18 mmol/l and represents the unmeasured negative charge on albumin, phosphate, sulphate, lactate and other organic acids. Normal anion gap acidosis occurs when there is increased bicarbonate loss (e.g. from the GI tract in ureterosigmoidostomy or in proximal renal tubular acidosis), or if there is HCl retention (e.g. distal renal tubular acidosis or ammonium chloride ingestion). In maple syrup urine disease branched chain keto acids accumulate increasing the anion gap. Similarly, in salicylate poisoning this exogenous acid contributes to the unmeasured anions resulting in an increased anion gap acidosis. In the nephrotic syndrome serum albumin is low and, therefore, its effective negative charge is less, resulting in a lowering of the anion gap.

38. A

Alport's syndrome is usually transmitted as an X-linked dominant trait. It is due to an abnormality of type IV collagen resulting in weakness of the basement membranes. These are glomerulopathy, sensorineural deafness and anterior lenticonus and retinitis pigmentosa. Cardiac conduction defects are not a feature of Alport's syndrome. Post transplant antiglomerular basement membrane disease complicates less than 5% of Alport syndrome renal transplants.

39. A D

Dialysis-related amyloidosis is due to deposition of beta 2 microglobulin as amyloid fibrils predominantly in and around joints classically resulting in carpal tunnel syndrome or shoulder girdle arthropathy. It can affect patients treated by all forms of dialysis. Transplantation results in increased beta 2 microglobulin excretion and improvement of the condition. There is no increase in renal transplant failure. It is not associated with any particular primary renal disease – diabetics are less likely to survive the long time on dialysis necessary for the condition to manifest itself.

40. Cyclosporin A

☐ A causes afferent arteriolar vasoconstriction

☐ B interferes with interleukin-2 gene transcription

☐ C toxicity can be due to allopurinol co-administration

☐ D causes glucose intolerance

☐ E causes gingival hyperplasia

Answers overleaf

40. A B E

Cyclosporin A exerts its immunosuppressive action by interference with interleukin-2 gene transcription by inhibition of calcineurin phosphatase. Vasoconstriction of the renal afferent arterioles reduces glomerular filtration rate and is a major side effect often necessitating dose reduction. Allopurinol blocks xanthine oxidase and increases azathioprine toxicity but does not interact with cyclosporin. Cyclosporin A has been used to treat early autoimmune type I diabetes to prolong the honeymoon period – it does not cause glucose intolerance (unlike FK506). It does cause gingival hyperplasia, particularly when used in combination with calcium antagonists.

ENDOCRINE AND METABOLIC MEDICINE

Mark your answers with a tick (True) or a cross (False) in the box provided. Leave the box blank for 'Don't know'.

41. The following may enhance the oral hypoglycaemic action of sulphonylureas:

☐ A trimethoprim

☐ B bendrofluazide

☐ C rifampicin

☐ D bezafibrate

☐ E alcohol

42. The following are causes of hyperprolactinaemia:

☐ A ranitidine

☐ B thyroxine

☐ C methyldopa

☐ D oestrogens

☐ E haloperidol

43. Adrenal insufficiency

☐ A can be precipitated by rifampicin

☐ B requires treatment with high dose steroids

☐ C does not require treatment with fludrocortisone

☐ D circulating adrenal antibodies occur in over 70%

☐ E can be associated with spastic paralysis in females

Answers overleaf

41. A D E

Rifampicin reduces the effect of sulphonylureas by accelerating metabolism via enzyme induction. Bendrofluazide, and other thiazide and loop diuretics, cause insulin resistance and glucose intolerance. Alcohol, sulphonamide antibiotics, trimethoprim, miconazole, fibrates and sulphinpyrazone enhance the effect of sulphonylureas.

42. C D E

H_2 blockade does not interfere with prolactin secretion but cimetidine (not ranitidine) is a cause of gynaecomastia. In normal physiological circumstances prolactin is under tonic inhibitory control by the dopaminergic system of the hypothalamus. Dopamine depleting agents (e.g. methyldopa) and dopamine receptor blockers (e.g. metoclopramide and haloperidol) result in increased prolactin release. Oestrogens which increase the number and activity of prolactin secreting cells do not act through dopamine related mechanisms. Hypothyroidism, via thyroid stimulating hormone, frequently causes increased prolactin which is suppressed by thyroxine.

43. A

Adrenal insufficiency can be due to many causes including tuberculosis, autoimmune adrenalitis, systemic fungal infection, metastatic carcinoma, HIV infection, antiphospholipid syndrome, amyloidosis and acute haemorrhage in sepsis such as meningococcaemia. Rifampicin is an enzyme inducer and can unmask adrenal insufficiency. Treatment is with the smallest dose of hydrocortisone or cortisone necessary to relieve the patient's symptoms in order to avoid the side effects of glucocorticoids. Fludrocortisone is necessary in a single daily dose of 50–200 µg depending on blood pressure, serum potassium and serum renin. Adrenal autoantibodies can be detected in 70% of patients with autoimmune adrenalitis but not the other causes. Adrenomyeloneuropathy is an X-linked recessive disorder of long chain fatty acid metabolism that is characterised by spastic paraparesis and adrenal failure in young men.

44. Glucocorticoid effects on bone metabolism include

- ☐ A increased osteoblastic activity
- ☐ B reduced gastrointestinal absorption of calcium
- ☐ C reduced 25-hydroxylation of vitamin D
- ☐ D reduced calcitonin levels
- ☐ E increased renal excretion of calcium

45. Hypocalciuric hypercalcaemia

- ☐ A is an X-linked recessive trait
- ☐ B occurs in the milk-alkali syndrome
- ☐ C is corrected by parathyroidectomy
- ☐ D is associated with pituitary tumours
- ☐ E is masked by thiazide diuretic use

46. Effects of drugs on thyroid function tests include

- ☐ A beta blockers can reduce T4
- ☐ B dopamine can reduce thyroid stimulating hormone (TSH)
- ☐ C amiodarone can reduce or increase TSH
- ☐ D lithium can reduce TSH
- ☐ E phenytoin can reduce T4

Answers overleaf

44. B E

Glucocorticoid-induced osteoporosis occurs as a result of increased osteoclast-mediated bone resorption and decreased osteoblast-mediated bone formation. Glucocorticoids also cause a decrease in intestinal absorption of both calcium and phosphate. In addition, renal excretion of calcium is increased probably due to a direct effect on tubular reabsorption of calcium. In addition, glucocorticoids cause a reduction in sex hormone production. There are no consistent abnormalities in vitamin D, PTH, or calcitonin levels.

45. None correct

Familial hypocalciuric hypercalcaemia is a relatively benign autosomal dominant disease. Although PTH levels may be elevated hypercalcaemia is not PTH dependent. There is an abnormality of the calcium-sensing receptor resulting in a shift in the calcium set point for PTH secretion from apparently otherwise normal glands. It is not associated with other (multiple) endocrine neoplasia. Thiazide diuretics can cause hypercalcaemia in patients with borderline hyperparathyroidism and are used as a treatment to reduce urinary calcium loss in idiopathic hypercalciuria.

46. B C E

Many drugs can affect thyroid function tests and results must be interpreted with caution in the ill patient and in those taking certain widely used drugs. Beta blockers, amiodarone and glucocorticoids reduce peripheral deiodination of T4 to T3. Dopamine has direct inhibitory effects on the pituitary to reduce TSH release. Amiodarone has complex effects on thyroid function as a result of its high iodine content and inhibition of peripheral deiodination. It can cause either hyper- or hypothyroidism. Lithium inhibits thyroid T4 and T3 release and may lead to increased TSH. Phenytoin, by hepatic enzyme induction, increases T4 metabolism.

47. Insulin resistance

- ☐ A is increased by doxasocin
- ☐ B is unaffected by beta blockade
- ☐ C is increased by thiazide diuretics
- ☐ D is associated with elevated high density lipoprotein
- ☐ E is reduced by angiotensin converting enzyme inhibitors

48. The syndrome of inappropriate antidiuretic hormone (SIADH) production

- ☐ A is a recognised complication of Guillain–Barré syndrome
- ☐ B can occur with lithium therapy
- ☐ C urine osmolality is typically less than 300 mosmol/l
- ☐ D aldosterone levels are suppressed
- ☐ E responds to demeclocycline

49. Steroid hormone receptors

- ☐ A interact with RNA to cause their effect
- ☐ B are located on the cell membrane
- ☐ C are similar to vitamin D receptors
- ☐ D are blocked by aminoglutethimide
- ☐ E are stabilised by heat shock proteins

50. Adrenal ll-beta hydroxylase deficiency

- ☐ A is a cause of virilisation in females
- ☐ B causes salt losing in infancy
- ☐ C is associated with hypertension
- ☐ D the principal urinary metabolites are 17 deoxysteroids
- ☐ E is autosomal recessive

Answers overleaf

47. C E

Insulin resistance is increased by treatment with beta blockers and thiazide diuretics. It is reduced by doxasocin and angiotensin converting enzyme inhibitors. The dyslipidaemia of insulin resistance is characterised by decreased HDL cholesterol, increased very low density lipoprotein triglyceride and increased low density lipoprotein cholesterol.

48. A D E

SIADH can be caused by a number of pathologies, including pituitary/intracranial disease, pulmonary lesions, Guillain–Barré syndrome and acute intermittent porphyria. Lithium is a cause of nephrogenic diabetes insipidus not SIADH. The urine osmolality is inappropriately high in relation to serum (which is usually less than 270 mosmol/l) and typically is in the range of 350–400 mosmol/l. Oedema does not occur because aldosterone secretion is suppressed, which in turn causes increased urinary sodium excretion. Demeclocycline is effective for chronic SIADH and acts by blocking the renal tubular effect of ADH.

49. C E

Steroid receptors represent a class of ligand activated transcription factors, with differing binding affinities that include vitamin D receptors and thyroid hormone receptors. They are located intracellularly and function primarily by virtue of their DNA binding activity. Certain steroid receptors are stabilised by heat shock proteins. Aminoglutethimide acts predominantly by inhibiting the conversion of androgens to oestrogens in the peripheral tissues.

50. A C E

Il-beta hydroxylose deficiency is an autosomal recessive condition causing congenital adrenal hyperplasia.The clinical features include hypertension and virilisation. The principal steroids excreted are androgens and II deoxycortisol metabolites. 21-hydroxylase deficiency, which also causes congenital adrenal hyperplasia, can present with salt wasting. Elevated urinary 17 deoxysteroids are seen in 21-hydroxylase deficiency.

RHEUMATOLOGY AND IMMUNOLOGY

Mark your answers with a tick (True) or a cross (False) in the box provided. Leave the box blank for 'Don't know'.

51. Hereditary angioedema

☐ A is inherited as a sex linked condition

☐ B can present with abdominal pain

☐ C is due to a deficiency in the C1q component of complement

☐ D results in low C2 and C4 complement components in plasma

☐ E responds to danazol treatment

52. Type IV hypersensitivity

☐ A involves mast cell degranulation

☐ B occurs in contact dermatitis

☐ C is initiated by antibody

☐ D can result in granulomatous reactions

☐ E is a feature of myasthenia gravis

53. Rheumatoid factors

☐ A are typically IgM antibodies

☐ B bind the Fab fragment of IgG

☐ C include antinuclear antibodies

☐ D are present in the synovial fluid in rheumatoid arthritis

☐ E are acute phase reactants

Answers overleaf

51. B D E

Hereditary angioedema is an autosomal dominant trait characterised by low (less than 25% of normal) to undetectable functional activity of C1 inhibitor. This deficiency of C1 inhibitor permits C1s to continuously cleave its substrates, C4 and C2, producing a secondary deficiency in these proteins. Clinically the illness is characterised by recurrent episodes of subcutaneous oedema, upper respiratory tract oedema/obstruction or abdominal pain due to bowel wall oedema. Treatment of an acute attack includes fresh plasma to restore C1 inhibitor levels and support therapy. Danazol is effective in reducing episodes of angioedema.

52. B D

Type IV hypersensitivity (delayed hypersensitivity) reactions are initiated by T cells not antibody. Histologically, delayed–type hypersensitivity reactions consist of infiltrating lymphocytes, macrophages and occasionally eosinophils. Mast cells are not involved in Type IV hypersensitivity but are pivotal in Type I sensitivity which results in mast cell degranulation. Chronic lesions can show granulomatous reactions as in tuberculosis. Contact dermatitis is a Type IV hypersensitivity reaction. Myasthenia gravis is an antibody mediated autoimmune disease of the neuromuscular junction (Type II hypersensitivity). Type III hypersensitivity is due to immune complex formation, as in serum sickness.

53. A D

Rheumatoid factors (RFs) are autoantibodies against the IgG Fc, not Fab, fragment. RFs are found in both the healthy population and several disease conditions including of course rheumatoid arthritis (50–90%) and SLE (15–35%). RFs of the IsM isotype are predominant in serum and have also been found in the synovial fluid of inflamed joints in rheumatoid arthritis. RFs are distinct from antinuclear antibodies and are not acute phase proteins although following infections and immunisations, RFs can be transiently produced in healthy subjects.

54. In methotrexate therapy

- ☐ A baseline liver biopsy is recommended if there is a history of heavy alcohol consumption
- ☐ B folic acid therapy reduces efficacy
- ☐ C NSAIDs increase toxicity
- ☐ D dose should be reduced in renal insufficiency
- ☐ E diabetes mellitus is a risk factor for hepatic toxicity

55. Side effects of gold therapy

- ☐ A are associated with HLA-DR4 antigen
- ☐ B include crescentic nephritis
- ☐ C thrombocytopenia is usually due to marrow suppression
- ☐ D interstitial pneumonitis is a late side effect
- ☐ E vasomotor reactions can be treated with angiotensin converting enzyme inhibitors

56. In scleroderma

- ☐ A vascular fibrosis is mediated by transforming growth factor-beta (TGF-β)
- ☐ B anti-RNA polymerase antibodies are associated with renal involvement
- ☐ C males and females are affected to the same extent
- ☐ D microangiopathic haemolytic anaemia can occur
- ☐ E hypertension should be treated with ACE inhibitors

Answers overleaf

54. A C D E

Methotrexate is a folate antagonist that is used to treat psoriasis, rheumatoid arthritis and non-renal vasculitis. The potential development of serious hepatic and pulmonary toxicity is the major concern. Other side effects include GI intolerance, stomatitis and bone marrow suppression. If there is a past history of heavy alcohol consumption or liver disease a baseline liver biopsy is recommended. Diabetes and obesity are risk factors for hepatic fibrosis. Methotrexate should be used with particular caution in the presence of renal insufficiency and drugs that alter the clearance of methotrexate, such as NSAIDs. Folic acid therapy can reduce side effects but does not alter efficacy.

55. D

Gold-induced proteinuria and thrombocytopenia occur more frequently in patients who possess HLA-DR3 antigens. Transient proteinuria, microscopic haematuria and nephrotic syndrome are well described complications of gold therapy. Renal biopsy usually reveals membranous nephropathy but minimal change disease has also been described. Crescentic nephritis may complicate treatment with penicillamine. The thrombocytopenia is usually due to immune destruction of platelets with an active marrow rather than marrow suppression. Interstitial pneumonitis can occur after a high cumulative dose (above 500 mg) and usually responds to withdrawal of gold and administration of systemic glucocorticoids. Vasomotor reactions are more frequent in patients receiving angiotensin converting enzyme inhibitors.

56. A B D E

The vascular fibrogenic response that characterises scleroderma is mediated by transforming growth factor-beta (TGF-β) in conjunction with platelet derived growth factor and basic fibroblast growth factor. Scleroderma renal crisis is frequent in patients with anti-RNA polymerase antibodies (24%) in contrast to those with anti-topoisomerase 1 antibodies (10%). Females are affected 3 times more frequently than males. The hypertension of scleroderma is mediated by activation of the renin-angiotensin system and should be treated by ACE inhibition. Diuretics which activate the renin-angiotensin system should be avoided as they can precipitate renal crisis.

57. Side effects of non steroidal anti inflammatory drugs (NSAIDs) include

☐ A nephrotic syndrome

☐ B hypokalaemia

☐ C *Helicobacter pylori*-related gastric ulceration

☐ D heart failure

☐ E hyponatraemia

58. In rheumatoid arthritis

☐ A there is an association with HLA DR3

☐ B activated T cells are present in the synovium

☐ C anti-tumour necrosis factor beta antibody can suppress disease activity

☐ D concordance in twin surveys is greater than 80%

☐ E chondrocytes express HLA class II antigens

59. Reiter's disease

☐ A is associated with HLA B27

☐ B antibodies to extractable nuclear antigen Jo1 develop

☐ C can follow infection with shigella

☐ D is more frequent in males

☐ E complicates gonococcal urethritis

60. Inherent complement deficiencies are associated with

☐ A membranoproliferative nephropathy

☐ B a lupus-like syndrome

☐ C recurrent meningitis

☐ D pancreatitis

☐ E X-linked transmission

Answers overleaf

57. A D E

Nephrotic syndrome with or without interstitial nephritis is a rare side effect of NSAIDs - particularly propionic acid derivatives. NSAIDs inhibit prostaglandin-mediated renin release resulting in hypoaldosteronism and consequent hyperkalaemia. NSAID-induced ulcers are not related to *H. pylori* infection, serological markers and biopsy evidence of gastric colonisation are no greater than in normal controls. NSAIDs antagonise the effects of arginine vasopressin which can result in either hyponatraemia or fluid retention which can precipitate heart failure.

58. B E

Rheumatoid arthritis is associated with HLA DR1and HLA DR4, but twin surveys reveal a concordance of less than 30%, suggesting a polygenic rather than single gene effect. There is evidence of B cell overactivity (rheumatoid factor, autoantibodies) and increased activated T cells in the peripheral blood and joints. Interleukin-I and tumour necrosis factor alpha are elevated in the joints and blockade of TNF-alpha with monoclonal antibody therapy reduces disease activity. Abnormal HLA class II expression or chondrocytes, fibroblasts and endothelial cells occur and are likely to be involved in antigen presentation to the T cell receptor.

59. A C D

Reiter's disease is a reactive arthritis secondary to infection – frequently dysentery or non-specific urethritis (not gonococcal). The disease is thought to be due to immune complex deposition but antibodies to nuclear antigens are not a feature. The disease usually affects males aged 16 to 35 years and is strongly associated with HLA B27. Other features of Reiter's disease include plantar fascitis, keratoderma blemorhagica and circinate balinitis.

60. B C

The genes for all the complement proteins are located in the major histocompatibility complex region of chromosome 6. Deficiencies are associated with lupus-like syndromes and recurrent bacterial infections, especially with encapsulated organisms such as meningococcus. Pancreatitis can lead to complement consumption and low circulating complement levels but is not a feature of inherited deficiencies. Membranoproliferative glomerulonephritis can result from an autoantibody to C3 – C3 nephritic factor.

Mark your answers with a tick (True) or a cross (False) in the box provided. Leave the box blank for 'Don't know'.

61. Internuclear ophthalmoplegia

- ☐ A results in failure of abduction of the eye ipsilateral to the lesion
- ☐ B when caused by lesions of the right side, causes nystagmus on abduction of the left eye
- ☐ C results from a lesion in the centre for lateral gaze
- ☐ D does not affect vertical gaze
- ☐ E causes dilation of the ipsilateral pupil

62. In multiple sclerosis

- ☐ A saltatory conduction is impaired
- ☐ B MHC class II expression is increased in the CNS
- ☐ C the blood–brain barrier is intact
- ☐ D oligodendrocytes are unaffected
- ☐ E helper T cells are found in acute lesions

63. Anti-acetylcholine antibodies

- ☐ A are typically IgM isotype
- ☐ B can result from penicillamine treatment
- ☐ C are polyclonal
- ☐ D may arise as a paraneoplastic phenomenon
- ☐ E are not complement fixing

Answers overleaf

61. B D

Internuclear ophthalmoplegia is a common brain stem lesion often resulting from demyelination. The lesion is in the medial longitudinal fasciculus and results in impaired adduction on the side of the lesion and nystagmus on abduction of the contralateral eye. It does not affect vertical gaze or the pupil.

62. A B E

Multiple sclerosis (MS) is an acquired defect of oligodendrocytes that are responsible for producing myelin. As a result of demyelination the normal saltatory conduction between nodes of Ranvier is impaired. In MS breakdown of the blood–brain barrier precedes both symptoms and MRI signs of demyelination. Perivascular helper T cells are found in acute MS lesions and there is abnormal MHC class II expression on macrophages and astrocytes resulting in antigen presentation and immune injury.

63. B C

Anti-acetylcholine receptor antibodies have a high sensitivity and specificity for myasthenia gravis. They are mainly IgG and can cross the feto-placental barrier. Their main pathogenic role is via complement dependent lysis of the post-synaptic membrane. Anti-acetylcholine receptor antibodies are of high affinity, idiotypically heterogenous and variable in antigenic specificity. They do not arise as a paraneoplastic phenomenon and do not occur in the Eaton–Lambert syndrome. Penicillamine can result in the development of antiacetylcholine receptor antibodies with or without development of myasthenia gravis.

64. The neuroleptic malignant syndrome

- ☐ A can occur with benzodiazepines
- ☐ B is frequently complicated by rhabdomyolysis
- ☐ C pyrexia is uncommon
- ☐ D may respond to bromocriptine
- ☐ E can complicate antiparkinsonian therapy

65. Beta interferon in multiple sclerosis

- ☐ A reduces relapse rate by 70%
- ☐ B inhibits MHC class II expression
- ☐ C improves blood–brain barrier integrity in active disease
- ☐ D short term use can exacerbate disease
- ☐ E increases suppressor T cell activity

66. Huntington's disease

- ☐ A neuronal degeneration results from apoptosis
- ☐ B is X-linked
- ☐ C is caused by an expansion of a polyglutamine trinucleotide repeat in the Huntington's gene
- ☐ D degeneration is primarily in the olive and Purkinje neurones
- ☐ E characteristically presents by age 40

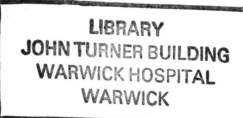
Answers overleaf

64. B D E

The neuroleptic malignant syndrome usually complicates phenothiazine therapy and often occurs within 2 weeks of a change of dose. It can be a complication of tricyclic antidepressants, levodopa and amantadine, and phenytoin. The classical features are hyperthermia and rigidity with autonomic dysfunction and altered state of consciousness in many. Rhabdomyolysis, seizures, DIC and catatonia frequently occur. Treatment is largely supportive with withdrawal of the neuroleptic, but dantrolene, bromocriptine and benzodiazepines have all been used with favourable effects.

65. B C D E

Beta interferon may influence the activity of multiple sclerosis (MS) through several mechanisms including down regulation of abnormal CNS HLA class II antigen expression, enhanced activity of suppressor T cells and inhibition of gamma interferon. In relapsing MS beta interferon reduces the clinical relapse rate by approximately 30%. Magnetic resonance scanning can document blood–brain barrier leakage in active disease and this has been shown to improve following beta interferon treatment. However, short term use (for less than 6 months) may exacerbate disease.

66. A C

Huntington's disease is an autosomal dominant neurodegenerative disorder characterised by variable age at onset (typically 45–65), uncontrolled movements, altered behaviour and cognitive decline. It is caused by expansion of a polyglutamine trinucleotide repeat in the coding region of the gene – the size of the expansion predicts age of onset. Neurodegeneration is primarily in the caudate and putamen by apoptosis. The spinocerebellar ataxias (which cause Purkinje and olive degeneration) are due to similar polyglutamine trinucleotide repeats in their respective genes. Trinucleotide repeat diseases are characteristically worse in each subsequent generation.

67. Progressive supranuclear palsy

- ☐ A is linked with apolipoprotein E polymorphism
- ☐ B responds to levodopa
- ☐ C is characterised by neurofibrillar tangles in the basal ganglia
- ☐ D is associated with dysphagia
- ☐ E is due to a primary mitochondrial DNA defect

68. Dystrophin

- ☐ A is abnormal in the limb girdle muscular dystrophies
- ☐ B binds to actin
- ☐ C is coded for by a gene on the X chromosome
- ☐ D is a transmembrane protein
- ☐ E is absent in Duchenne muscular dystrophy

69. Eaton–Lambert syndrome

- ☐ A is due to autoantibodies that bind to voltage-gated calcium channels
- ☐ B plasma exchange is an effective treatment
- ☐ C is associated with ventricular tachycardia
- ☐ D typically complicates pancreatic carcinoma
- ☐ E is associated with cerebellar degeneration

70. Apolipoprotein E

- ☐ A is not present in normal brain
- ☐ B is associated with mobilisation of cholesterol in tissue repair and growth
- ☐ C is encoded on chromosome 19
- ☐ D polymorphic variants are associated with Alzheimer's disease
- ☐ E is metabolised to an amyloid precursor protein

Answers overleaf

67. C D

Progressive supranuclear palsy presents with postural instability and falls, a levodopa-unresponsive Parkinsonian-like syndrome, vertical supranuclear palsy, dysarthria, dysphagia and frontal lobe abnormalities. It is not linked with apolipoprotein E (unlike Alzheimer's disease) or a mitochondrial DNA lesion. It is characterised by abundant neurofibrillar tangles in the basal ganglia and brain stem.

68. B C E

Dystrophin is a large submembrane protein that is orientated parallel to the muscle cell membranes and provides part of the extracellular to intracellular protein chain by linking beta-dystroglycan and F-actin. It is absent in Duchenne muscular dystrophy which is an X-linked disease. Limb girdle muscular dystrophies encompass a diverse set of diseases frequently associated with mutations to dystrophin associated proteins that interact with dystrophin (but not abnormalities of dystrophin itself).

69. A B

Eaton–Lambert myasthenic syndrome is an autoimmune paraneoplastic phenomenon secondary to antibodies against voltage-gated calcium channels (VGCC) expressed by the tumour (typically small cell lung cancer) that react with VGCC at the presynaptic level of neuromuscular cholinergic synapses. The syndrome usually responds to treatment of the underlying malignancy. It does not cause ventricular arrthymias or cerebellar degeneration.

70. B C D

Apoprotein E is a lipoprotein involved in the mobilisation of cholesterol for repair and growth. It is also produced by astrocytes and helps maintain myelin and neuronal membranes. The gene for Apo E is on chromosome 19 and has three common polymorphic variants – one of which, E4, is associated with Alzheimer's disease. As Apo E is found within the amyloid plaques associated with Alzheimer's disease it may be involved in the pathogenesis of this form of dementia. Amyloid precursor protein is distinct from apoprotein E.

Mark your answers with a tick (True) or a cross (False) in the box provided. Leave the box blank for 'Don't know'.

71. The following vaccines should be avoided in immuno-compromised patients:

- ☐ A diphtheria
- ☐ B BCG
- ☐ C hepatitis B
- ☐ D tetanus
- ☐ E pneumococcus

72. In schistosomiasis

- ☐ A risk of infection is related to fresh water exposure
- ☐ B nephrotic syndrome is a late sequelae
- ☐ C adult schistosomes multiply with a doubling rate of 28 days in the human host
- ☐ D eosinophilia does not occur
- ☐ E treatment with praziquantel should be continued for 6 weeks

73. *Borrelia burgdorferi*

- ☐ A is a spirochaete
- ☐ B causes babesiosis
- ☐ C characteristically causes erythema migrans
- ☐ D is resistant to penicillins
- ☐ E is Gram negative

Answers overleaf

71. B

Live vaccines should not be given to individuals with impaired immune response, whether caused by disease or as a result of radiotherapy, corticosteroids, or other immunosuppressive drugs. Diphtheria, hepatitis B, tetanus and pneumococcal vaccine are all inactive vaccines and are safe in immunosuppressed patients. Immunogenicity of vaccines, however, may be reduced in the immunosuppressed patient – this particularly applies to hepatitis B. Polyvalent pneumococcal polysaccharide vaccine is recommended for the immunisation of all immunosuppressed patients. Bacillus Calmette–Guerin vaccine is a live attenuated vaccine that can cause serious mycobacterial disease in the immunocompromised. Other live vaccines include yellow fever, measles, mumps, rubella and (Sabin) polio.

72. A B

Schistosomiasis is endemic in many areas of the Middle East, Africa, South America and Asia. The risk of infection is directly related to exposure to fresh water containing the intermediate snail hosts. Acute infection often produces an urticarial rash and is associated with eosinophilia. The adult schistosomes usually have a life span of 3 to 5 years and do not multiply in the human host. Pathology is caused by the immunological reaction to the deposited ova which causes an intense fibrotic reaction. Treatment with praziquantel at 40 mg/kg in a single oral dose is safe and effective.

73. A C E

Borrelia burgdorferi is a Gram-negative microaerophilic spirochaete that requires various vertebrate and arthropod hosts for survival. It is the causative organism of Lyme disease which usually begins with flu-like or meningitis-like symptoms accompanied by a characteristic rash, erythema migrans, at the site of the tick bite. After days to weeks, the spirochaete often disseminates from the skin and can affect multiple organ systems, most commonly the joints, nervous system and heart. *B. burgdorferi* is sensitive to penicillins and treatment of choice is amoxycillin or doxycycline. Babesiosis is a tick borne protozoan disease characterised by an acute febrile illness with haemolytic anaemia as a result of multiplication of the organisms in RBCs.

74. The systemic inflammatory response syndrome

☐ A is usually due to exotoxins released from Gram-positive bacteria

☐ B is mediated by tumour necrosis factor

☐ C can result in amyloidosis

☐ D is associated with tachypnoea

☐ E frequently complicates pancreatitis

75. Cryptococcal meningitis

☐ A can present with progressive dementia

☐ B CSF cryptococcal capsular antigen assay has a high sensitivity

☐ C amphotericin B is ineffective

☐ D frequently has associated choroidoretinitis

☐ E is associated with lymphoma

76. Vancomycin resistant enterococci

☐ A remain sensitive to aminoglycosides

☐ B spread by the faecal–oral route

☐ C renal failure is a risk factor

☐ D are always invasive

☐ E rapidly break down vancomycin

Answers overleaf

74. B D E

The systemic inflammatory response syndrome is a widespread inflammatory response to a variety of severe clinical insults including Gram-negative sepsis, pancreatitis, ischaemia-reperfusion injury. Exotoxins released from Gram-positive bacteria can induce the syndrome but this occurs much less frequently that with Gram-negative bacteria endotoxaemia. The principal cytokine mediators of the syndrome are tumour necrosis factor and interleukin-1.

75. A B E

Symptoms in cryptococcal meningitis are often more subtle than in classical bacterial meningitis. Cognitive impairment and progressive dementia may be present for months before diagnosis. The best diagnostic CSF tests are India ink and cryptococcal antigen, as other parameters are often normal. *Cryptococcus neoformans* is sensitive to a number of antifungals including amphotericin B. Choroidoretinitis is a feature of cytomegalovirus and toxoplasmosis but rarely occurs in cryptococcal infection alone. There is an increased risk of cryptococcal infection in patients on corticosteroids or who are immunosuppressed (e.g. lymphoma, organ transplantation, sarcoidosis or HIV infection).

76. B C

Vancomycin-resistant enterococci (VRE) make a set of enzymes that modify the peptidoglycan binding site that vancomycin normally binds to block cell wall synthesis, thereby inhibiting its binding and action. They do not rapidly metabolise vancomycin. Risk factors for VRE include length of hospital stay, immunosuppression, severity of illness, treatment with multiple antibiotics and renal failure. The organisms are spread by the faecal–oral route and frequently colonise patients without causing disease. They are, however, also highly resistant to penicillin and to aminoglycosides.

77. *Escherichia coli* 0157:H7

- ☐ A is a cause of pseudomembranous colitis
- ☐ B has an incubation period of 12 hours
- ☐ C is usually spread by the faecal–oral route
- ☐ D produces a shigella-like toxin
- ☐ E is associated with haemolytic uraemic syndrome

78. Concerning botulism

- ☐ A the causative organism is a Gram-negative rod
- ☐ B the toxin is usually detected in patient sera
- ☐ C it interferes with acetylcholine release
- ☐ D post-tetanic compound muscle action potentials are enhanced
- ☐ E it rarely causes ophthalmoplegia

79. Pneumococci

- ☐ A adhere to type II pneumocytes
- ☐ B serotyping is determined by cell wall antigens
- ☐ C induce tumour necrosis factor release
- ☐ D cell wall components are chemotaxic
- ☐ E are readily phagocytosed by polymorphonuclear cells

Answers overleaf

77. A D E

Escherichia coli 0157:H7 has emerged as a major cause of bloody diarrhoea and a causative organism of the haemolytic-uraemic syndrome. The organism adheres to the colonic mucosal surfaces and produces one or more shigella-like toxins that induce a haemorrhage colitis, pseudo membranes may be present. The toxin can initiate the haemolytic-uraemic syndrome if it gains access to the circulation. The majority of infection arises from transmission of the organism through the consumption of undercooked infected ground beef. The incubation period is typically 3 to 4 days.

78. C D

Ophthalmoparesis, facial weakness and bulbar palsy are the most frequent initial symptoms of botulism. Limb weakness and respiratory compromise may follow. The disease is caused by a toxin synthesised by *Clostridium botulinum*, a Gram-positive rod. The toxin impedes the formation of functioning acetylcholine vesicles thereby producing a presynaptic neuromuscular block. Post-tetanic potentiation of the compound muscle action potential, due to increased calcium mediated acetylcholine release, is a hallmark of presynaptic lesions. In affected patients only 35% have detectable toxin in their serum, stool specimens are more likely to be diagnostic.

79. A C D

Pneumococci are a major cause of pneumonia, empyaemia, otitis media, septicaemia and meningitis. The mucosal epithelium of the nasopharynx is the primary site of colonisation and subsequently pneumococci gain access to the lung by aspiration where they adhere to type II pneumocytes. The capsular polysaccharide protects pneumococci from phagocytosis and is the basis of serotyping, cell wall components induce the production of cytokines, including TNF, and initiate the inflammatory response by enchancing leucocyte recruitment. Resolution of pneumococcal infection begins when anticapsular antibodies opsonise the pneumococci and facilitate phagocytosis by polymorphonuclear cells.

80. *Listeria monocytogenes*

☐ A is a Gram-positive anaerobe

☐ B infection rates are increased in pregnancy

☐ C induces host-cell actin assembly

☐ D is resistant to phagocytosis

☐ E requires listerolysis O for pathogenecity

80. B C E

Listeria monocytogenes is an aerobic Gram-positive bacillus that is ubiquitous in the environment. Infection with this micro-organism is increased in the elderly, immunocompromised and pregnant (x 17 relative risk). *Listeria monocytogenes* is readily phagocytosed but has an enzyme – listerolysis O – an exotoxin that lyses the cell membrane of the phagolysosome and allows the organism to escape into the cytoplasm. Listeria exploit the host-cell contractile system for locomotion and cell-to-cell spread by promoting actin assembly that propels the micro-organism.

GASTROENTEROLOGY

Mark your answers with a tick (True) or a cross (False) in the box provided. Leave the box blank for 'Don't know'.

81. Alpha interferon treatment of hepatitis B

☐ A is most effective in patients with normal transaminase levels

☐ B results in long term remission in 80% of patients

☐ C is ineffective if there is coincidental hepatitis D infection

☐ D increases the risk of bacterial infections

☐ E frequently results in transient increases in transaminase levels

82. Hepatitis C

☐ A is a DNA virus

☐ B is a more frequent cause of chronic viral hepatitis than hepatitis B

☐ C often results in markedly elevated transaminases with only minor histological changes

☐ D does not respond to alpha interferon

☐ E can result in cryoglobulinaemic mesangiocapillary glomerulonephritis

83. Intestinal fat absorption

☐ A requires bile salt acids

☐ B occurs predominantly in the terminal ileum

☐ C requires pancreatic amylase

☐ D is inhibited by neomycin

☐ E requires a functional LDL receptor

Answers overleaf

81. D E

Alpha interferon treatment is indicated in patients with chronic hepatitis secondary to hepatitis B if there is persistent elevation of serum transaminases, detection of HBs Ag, Hbe Ag and HBV DNA in serum, chronic hepatitis in liver biopsy and compensated liver disease. A course of 4–6 months' treatment induces remission in 25% to 40% of patients. Patients with normal transaminase levels rarely respond to treatment. Transient increases in serum transaminase levels are common during therapy, especially in those in whom HBe Ag disappears. Other side effects include increased risks of bacterial infections, influenza-like reactions, chronic fatigue syndrome, autoimmune diseases and severe depression. Hepatitis D is responsive to alpha interferon but is more resistant than HBV and therefore higher doses are required.

82. B E

Hepatitis C is an RNA virus. The rate of chronic viral hepatitis in patients with acute hepatitis C is in the region of 80–100%. Hepatitis C is the most common cause of chronic viral hepatitis in the western world. Severe hepatitis can be present despite normal serum transaminase levels. The benefit of alpha interferon was demonstrated in non A non B hepatitis even before the discovery of HCV. Patients with HCV can develop vasculitis, cryoglobulinaemia and mesangiocapillary glomerulonephritis.

83. A D

Intestinal fat absorption is dependent on bile salt acids. These are detergents that emulsify coarse dietary fat globules leaving the stomach. Following this, pancreatic lipases break down the droplets leading to the formation of much smaller mixed micelles. Fatty acids, monoglycerides, phospholipids and cholesterol enter the enterocytes from the mixed micelles in the jejunum. Bile salt acids are reabsorbed in the terminal ileum. Neomycin owes its hypocholesterolaemic action to disruption of mixed micelles. The LDL receptor is not required for cholesterol absorption.

84. **Primary sclerosing cholangitis**

- ☐ A is associated with antineutrophil cytoplasmic antibodies
- ☐ B about two-thirds of patients are female
- ☐ C ursodeoxycholic acid improves survival
- ☐ D more frequently complicates ulcerative colitis than Crohn's disease
- ☐ E can recur following liver transplantation

85. **In haemochromatosis**

- ☐ A there is a mutation on chromosome 6
- ☐ B disease is more marked in heterozygotes with maternally transmitted mutations
- ☐ C gene-tracking can be undertaken on the basis of HLA-A type
- ☐ D the carrier frequency is 1:1000
- ☐ E heterozygotes usually develop liver failure above the age of 60

86. *Helicobacter pylori*

- ☐ A do not predispose to an increased risk of gastric lymphoma
- ☐ B produce ammonia
- ☐ C are Gram-positive rods
- ☐ D infection is frequently asymptomatic
- ☐ E should be irradicated in reflux oesophagitis

Answers overleaf

84. A D

Primary sclerosing cholangitis is a chronic progressive cholestatic liver disease characterised by continuing inflammation, necrosis and obliteration of intrahepatic and extrahepatic ducts. Approximately 75% of patients have inflammatory bowel disease (87% ulcerative colitis; 13% Crohn's disease) and two-thirds are male. It is associated with perinuclear antineutrophil cytoplasmic antibodies in a minority of cases. Ursodeoxycholic acid significantly improves the results of biochemical tests but does not improve symptoms, histological findings or prognosis. The disease usually progresses and results in cirrhosis, portal hypertension, and liver failure, ultimately necessitating liver transplantation. Sclerosing cholangitis does not recur post-transplant.

85. A C

Haemochromatosis is transmitted as an autosomal recessive trait. Heterozygotes rarely develop complications from iron overload but do have higher serum iron and transferrin saturation values than normal subjects. The responsible gene is tightly linked to the HLA class I region on chromosome 6. HLA-A typing therefore allows gene tracking through affected pedigrees. The carrier frequency is between 1 in 10–15 in Europeans.

86. B D

Helicobacter pylori is a microaerophilic Gram-negative rod. *H. pylori* colonise the stomach in at least a third of the world's human population. These organisms are urease positive and can therefore produce ammonia which is thought to result in epithelial damage. *H. pylori* infection is often asymptomatic but can result in peptic ulcer disease, gastritis, gastric carcinoma and gastric lymphoma. Helicobacter irradication is not recommended for reflux oesophagitis.

87. Gastric secretion

☐ A is inhibited by sympathetic nervous activation

☐ B is approximately 1 litre/day

☐ C is inhibited by low gastric pH

☐ D has a potassium concentration of 4 mmol/l

☐ E has a chloride concentration of 140 mmol/l

88. In polyposis coli

☐ A polyps typically develop above the age of 35 years

☐ B risk of colonic cancer is 50%

☐ C the gene has variable penetrance

☐ D duodenal polyps do not occur

☐ E the mutated gene is a tumour suppressor gene

89. In primary biliary cirrhosis

☐ A anti-mitochondrial antibodies correlate with severity

☐ B there is an association with HLA DR3

☐ C renal tubular acidosis develops due to copper deposition

☐ D lipoprotein(a) is elevated

☐ E familial cases are rare

Answers overleaf

87. A C E

Gastric secretion is stimulated by the vagus nerve, gastrin and histamine (therefore reduced by H_2 blockade); it is inhibited by sympathetic nervous activation, low gastric pH and small intestine inhibitory peptides (cholecystokinine-pancreazimin, GIP). Approximately 3 litres of gastric secretions are produced per day with a concentration profile of approximately hydrogen 100 mmol/l, sodium 50 mmol/l potassium 15 mmol/l, chloride 140 mmol/l and bicarbonate 15 mmol/l.

88. E

Familial adenomatous polyposis is an autosomal dominant disease with complete penetrance characterised by the presence of hundreds to thousands of colonic adenomatous polyps. Polyps occur at an average age of 15; all affected persons exhibit polyps by age 35. Colonic cancer is inevitable, unless the colon is removed, at an average age of 39 years. The adenomatous polyposis coli gene on chromosome 5 codes for a tumour suppressor protein involved in cell adhesion and regulation of cell growth. Gastric polyps occur in 50% and duodenal polyps in 90% of individuals – the lifetime risk of duodenal malignancy is 10%.

89. C

Anti-mitochondrial antibodies are found in 95% of patients with primary biliary cirrhosis and have a high specificity for this disorder but do not correlate with disease severity. Familial cases are common – prevalence in families with an affected member is 1000 times the general population. There is a weak association with HLA DR8; autoimmune hepatitis is associated with HLA B8 and DR3. Biochemical abnormalities include elevated serum caeruloplasmin levels and copper deposition in the kidney leading to renal tubular acidosis. Serum lipids are elevated but lipoprotein(a) is reduced and atherosclerotic risk is not increased.

90. Respiratory complications of parenteral nutrition include

☐ A type II respiratory failure

☐ B pneumothorax

☐ C pulmonary abcess

☐ D impaired respiratory muscle function

☐ E pulmonary embolism

90. A B C D E

Complications of parenteral nutrition can include those related to central venous cannulation such as pneumothorax or haemothorax, thrombosis, embolism, septicaemia and metastatic infection. Metabolic complications, related to the composition of the i.v. feed, include respiratory failure due to excessive carbohydrate load and CO_2 production, and hypophosphataemia resulting in muscle weakness. These complications usually arise in patients with underlying pulmonary disease but can prolong the need for intermittent positive pressure ventilation. Other metabolic complications include hyper- and hypoglycaemia, hyperosmolar coma, acid–base disturbance, fatty liver, hepatic encephalopathy and deficiency disorders. Effects on the gut include brush border atrophy, increased permeability and an exaggerated splanchnic response to endotoxin.

MOLECULAR MEDICINE

Mark your answers with a tick (True) or a cross (False) in the box provided. Leave the box blank for 'Don't know'.

91. The complement system

- ☐ A can only be activated by immunoglobulins
- ☐ B involves a cascade of proteins resulting in formation of the membrane attack complex
- ☐ C is involved in tissue injury in lupus nephritis
- ☐ D is controlled by membrane bound proteins that inactivate the terminal complement components
- ☐ E is defective in paroxsymal nocturnal haemoglobinuria

92. Mitochondrial DNA

- ☐ A is single stranded
- ☐ B abnormalities are associated with diabetes mellitus
- ☐ C is paternally inherited
- ☐ D consists of 23 molecules per mitochondria
- ☐ E mutates more frequently than nuclear DNA

93. The polymerase chain reaction

- ☐ A produces multiple copies of DNA
- ☐ B occurs at 40°C
- ☐ C requires oligonucleotide primers
- ☐ D can be used to detect functional polymorphisms
- ☐ E is of high specifity but low sensitivity

Answers overleaf

91. B C D E

The complement system amplifies the action of antibodies which activate complement component 1 – the classical pathway – but microbial polysaccharides can also directly activate component 3 – the alternative pathway. The consequence of activation is the assembly of the late complement components into the membrane attack complex that punches holes in the cell membrane. Complement activation has been implicated in tissue injury in a wide variety of circumstances including inflammation and ischaemia. In the normal situation, injury to human cells is reduced by inactivation of the terminal components by membrane bound complement control proteins. These control proteins are defective in paroxysmal nocturnal haemoglobinuria.

92. B E

Mitochondrial DNA is a double stranded, circular molecule that mutates over ten times more frequently than nuclear DNA. Each mitochondrion contains 2–10 DNA molecules. It has no introns nor an effective repair system and therefore a random mutation will usually strike a coding DNA sequence. Mitochondrial DNA is maternally inherited. Classic mitochondrial DNA diseases include Leber's optic atrophy, chronic progressive external ophthalmoplegia and mitochondrial myopathy. Systemic features of mitochondrial DNA mutations include diabetes mellitus, cardiomyopathy, lactic acidosis, Fanconi's syndrome and Wolff–Parkinson–White syndrome.

93. A C D

The polymerase chain reaction amplifies DNA that has first been separated into single strands by heat. Two oligonucleotide primers are then used to bind to either side of the specific areas of interest of the DNA and a polymerase enzyme catalyses the synthesis of a copy of the nucleotide sequence between the primers. The process can be repeated many times to make multiple copies of the specific gene of interest. The technique can be used to detect differences in genes – polymorphisms, presence of foreign genetic material and even RNA from either messenger RNA or RNA viruses using reverse transcriptase. The technique is highly specific for the oligonucleotide sequence used in the primers and is also of high sensitivity – contamination with only a single DNA copy can lead to false-positive results unless rigorous controls are used.

94. The LDL receptor

- ☐ A is restricted to the cell surface of tissues
- ☐ B catalyses HDL at a lower rate that LDL
- ☐ C is defective in familial hypercholesterolaemia
- ☐ D mediates down regulation of HMG CoA reductase
- ☐ E is encoded on the X chromosome

95. Adhesion molecule interactions

- ☐ A can be homophilic
- ☐ B are present at adherens junctions
- ☐ C require beta 2 microglobulin
- ☐ D can occur via the RGD motif
- ☐ E rarely result in signal transduction

96. The P53 gene

- ☐ A is frequently mutated in lung cancer
- ☐ B inhibits apoptosis
- ☐ C is induced by alcohol
- ☐ D develops specific mutations in response to tobacco smoke carcinogens
- ☐ E suppresses tumour growth

Answers overleaf

94. C D

The LDL receptor continuously recycles from the cell surface to endosomes (or receptorsomes),internalising LDL for catabolism. HDL does not compete with LDL for receptor mediated uptake. Once internalised LDL undergoes lysosomal degradation and its cholesterol ester is hydrolysed to free cholesterol. Release of this free cholesterol from the lysosome regulates cellular cholesterol content by:

- down regulating 3-hydroxy-3-methyl glutaryl-CoA (HMG-CoA) reductase
- repressing LDL receptor synthesis
- activating acyl CoA: cholesterol O-acetyl-transferase (ACAT) so that any cholesterol surplus to requirements is reconverted to cholesterol ester and stored as droplets in the cytoplasm.

The LDL receptor is encoded on chromosome 19 and more than 100 mutations occurring in the genes encoding this receptor-mediated LDL catabolism can lead to the clinical syndrome of familial hyper-cholesterolaemia. Familial hypercholesterolaemia is autosomal, affecting males and females equally and therefore the LDL receptor could not be encoded on the X chromosome.

95. A B D

Adhesion molecules include the integrins, immunoglobulin superfamily, cadherins and selectins. They orchestrate cell–cell and cell–matrix interactions and as such are involved in a wide range of processes including embryogenesis, inflammatory reactions and wound repair. Several adhesion molecules (including cadherins and platelet-endothelial cell adhesion molecule – PECAM) can bind to an identical molecule on another cell (homophilic adhesion). Cadherins establish molecular links between adjacent cells at adherens junctions. The integrins recognise the amino acid sequence arginine–glycerine–aspartic acid (RGD) motif present in the extracellular matrix. Signal transduction follows adhesion molecule interaction and affects many processes inside the cell including proliferation, secretion and apoptosis. Beta 2 microglobulin is not an adhesion molecule – it is part of the HLA system.

96. A D E

P53 is a tumour suppressor gene that regulates apoptosis and can halt the cell cycle in response to cell injury. The frequency of P53 mutations is 90% in small cell and 55% in non small cell lung cancer. Retroviral mediated wild type P53 gene transfer to tumours of patients with lung cancer increases apoptosis and tumour regression. Tobacco smoke carcinogens induce a specific pattern of P53 mutations and detection of P53 mutations in sputum can precede diagnosis of lung cancer. Cytochrome P450 (not P53) is induced by alcohol and enzyme inducing drugs.

97. The helper T cell receptor interacts with

- ☐ A HLA class II antigen
- ☐ B CD3
- ☐ C HLA class I antigen
- ☐ D processed antigen
- ☐ E beta 2 microglobulin

98. Antisense oligonucleotides

- ☐ A consist of 13 to 20 amino acids
- ☐ B hybridise with native DNA to reduce gene expression
- ☐ C lead to expression of 'nonsense' proteins
- ☐ D block transcription factors
- ☐ E increase messenger RNA degradation

99. Tumour necrosis factor-alpha

- ☐ A is predominantly synthesised by activated T cells
- ☐ B circulates bound to soluble receptors
- ☐ C predominantly acts in a paracrine fashion
- ☐ D is released in response to endotoxin stimulation
- ☐ E promotes fibrotic reactions

100. Nuclear factor kB

- ☐ A binds to cytoplasmic proteins
- ☐ B activates tumour necrosis factor-alpha
- ☐ C regulates the expression of inflammatory response genes
- ☐ D is inhibited by glucocorticoids
- ☐ E enhances inducible nitric oxide synthase

Answers overleaf

97. A D

The T cell receptor complex recognises processed antigen in the context of major histocompatability complex class I or II antigens depending on the type of T cells. Helper cells recognise antigen with class II and supressor/cytotoxic T cells recognize antigen with class I. CD3 is closely associated with the T cell receptor and is responsible for transducing the antigen recognition signal into the T cell. Beta 2 microglobulin is part of HLA class I.

98. E

Antisense oligonucleotides have a deoxynucleotide sequence of 13 to 20 base pairs in length – not amino acids. They hybridise to a specific complementary mRNA sequence, which is then subject to RNAse degradation resulting in a translational block. They do not lead to expression of 'nonsense' proteins. Decoy oligonucleotides (not antisense oligonucleotides) mimic the DNA binding domain of certain transcription factors and thereby down regulate gene expression.

99. B C D

Tumour necrosis factor-alpha is a proinflammatory cytokine, predominantly synthesised by macrophages and released in response to bacterial or inflammatory stimuli. It predominantly acts in a paracrine fashion at the site of release to promote inflammation/ injury rather than repair or fibrosis. It has two receptors present on the surface of nearly all cells, except erythrocytes, and cleaved fragments of these receptors act as binding proteins in the serum.

100. A B C D E

Nuclear factor kB is a transcription factor that acts on genes for pro-inflammatory cytokines (TNF, IL-1E, IL-2, IL-6), chemokines, enzymatic mediators of inflammation, immune receptors and adhesion molecules. It therefore has a pivotal role in the inflammatory response. In unstimulated cells it is found in the cytoplasm bound to a carrier. On activation it passes into the nucleus to act on specific promotor regions of target genes. Its actions are inhibited by glucocorticoids. Inducible nitric oxide synthase expression is enhanced by NF-kB.

BASIC SCIENCE REVISION CHECKLIST

Physiology

☐ Changes in pregnancy

☐ Haemoglobin function

☐ Physiology of bone

☐ Aetiology of oedema

Pathology

☐ Amyloid plaques

Hormone and mediator biochemistry

☐ Atrial natriuretic peptides

☐ Insulin/insulin resistance

☐ Adenosine

☐ ADH

☐ Aldosterone

☐ Angiotensin

☐ EDRF (nitric oxide)

☐ H_2 receptors

☐ Neurotransmitters

☐ Prostacyclin

☐ Somatostatin

☐ Steroid receptors

Miscellaneous

☐ Apolipoproteins

☐ Alpha$_1$-antitrypsin

☐ Mitochondrial DNA function

☐ Oncogenes

PHARMACOLOGY: REVISION CHECKLIST

Interactions/dose adjustment

☐ Drug interactions

☐ Pregnancy/breast feeding

☐ Dose adjustment in renal failure

☐ Adverse effects - general

Specific side-effects of drugs

☐ Causing hypothyroidism

☐ Asthma exacerbation

☐ Convulsions

☐ Gynaecomastia

☐ Hepatic enzyme inducers

☐ Hypokalaemia

Fundamental pharmacology

☐ Mechanisms of drug/antibiotic action

Most frequently considered individual agents

☐ Antipsychotics/depressants

☐ ACE inhibitors

☐ Amiodarone

☐ Digoxin

☐ Thiazides

☐ Anti-convulsants

☐ Sulphasalazine

Other 'topical' agents

☐ Azidothymidine (AZT)

☐ Gentamicin

☐ HMG Co-A reductase inhibitor

☐ L-dopa

☐ Lithium

☐ Penicillamine

☐ Warfarin

REVISION INDEX

Numbers refer to question numbers.

MOLECULAR MEDICINE